GOODBYE

ADRENAL FATIGUE!

THE ULTIMATE SOLUTION FOR ADRENAL FATIGUE & ADRENAL BURNOUT

ADRENAL DIET - HORMONE RESET - BALANCE HORMONES

Third Edition

SCOTT STERLING

© 2016

COPYRIGHT NOTICE

DISCLAIMER

Although the author and publisher have made every effort to ensure that the information in this book was correct at press time, the author and publisher do not assume and hereby disclaim any liability to any party for any loss, damage, or disruption caused by errors or omissions, whether such errors or omissions result from negligence, accident, or any other cause.

This book is not intended as a substitute for the medical advice of physicians. The reader should regularly consult a physician in matters relating to his/her health and particularly with respect to any symptoms that may require diagnosis or medical attention.

TABLE OF CONTENTS

INTRODUCTION

At some point in your life, regardless of what type of lifestyle you may be living now, you may find yourself feeling run down, tired, even exhausted with no visible or easily identifiable reason. Whilst some such symptoms can be attributed to a variety of factors – some lifestyle related and some related to identifiable medical conditions – some people are of the view that a condition known as adrenal fatigue could be an underlying cause, and is an issue of increasing importance. This relates to the work which is done by your adrenal glands, and whether, if they are not working to full capacity, this can result in you not feeling 100%.

For those who support the theory, adrenal fatigue is an amazingly common condition that affects millions of people worldwide, even though there is an assertion that it is taking time for medical science to recognize adrenal fatigue as a genuine and treatable syndrome. The view is taken that so many people are affected by these issues that the medical establishment is beginning to pay more attention to the condition, and is becoming increasingly concerned, with some even devoting their entire practice to the study and treatment of adrenal fatigue. Certainly it does stand to reason that, in the modern world – hectic and fast moving as it is – if there are new avenues to be explored to explain why an individual may feel increasingly tired, perhaps more susceptible to coughs and colds, together with a less clear mental pattern (for example, a shorter temper or memory) – then these need to be explored further, and if this might seem to describe some of the symptoms you are experiencing, then this book can help you to do just that.

In spite of the fact that it is now becoming better known, this condition is not as easily identifiable as you might expect, with some people experiencing symptoms thought to be related to adrenal fatigue for years without ever realizing that it exists. This book is designed to help as many people as possible recognize the signs that they may be among that number, and to offer options which can help improve both health related to the adrenal glands, and more generally.

This book is designed to give you the information you need to determine if you are one of the millions who are thought to suffer from this affliction, and if you think that you are, the book further equips you with the tools you need to begin your journey to recovery, and prevent the necessity of treatment. We will look at the following:

- What are the adrenal glands? What do they do and why is this important?

- What is Adrenal Fatigue? How is it categorized?

- What are thought to be the underlying causes of Adrenal Fatigue?

- What lifestyle changes can be employed to recover from Adrenal Fatigue? What role can exercise, diet and routine play?

The goal of this book is to give you the tools to help you understand the condition, consider whether or not you need to seek medical attention, and set yourself on a path to self treatment and complete recovery. Even in broader terms, if you have ever felt that you may be somewhat low on energy, then we urge you to read this book , and put its advice into practical, daily use. The thoughts presented in this book include options around the three key pillars of stress, diet and exercise. These can sometimes be linked to each other, but all underpin a well constituted and healthy mind and body – this means that any actions which can be taken to improve how an individual deals with stress, and how they can improve their diet and exercise regime to achieve those goals are likely to contribute to wider health, as well as ensuring better functioning adrenal glands. Whilst there are no guarantees, many of the simple actions and pieces of advice in the book can help underpin a healthier lifestyle more generally – the vast majority of the actions are simple, and you may even have tried a few of them before. In addition, they are things which allow you to take control of your own situation - there's really nothing to lose.

CHAPTER 1: ADRENAL GLANDS - WHAT ARE THEY, AND WHY ARE THEY IMPORTANT?

The first thing we have to explore is what the adrenal glands are, where they sit in your body, and what are the key functions that they undertake. To understand this is to better understand why they are so important, and why anything which can affect how efficient they are needs to be explored.

What are the Adrenal Glands?

Your adrenal glands are about the size of a walnut, and each of them sits atop one of your kidneys; in fact, the word "adrenal" could be literally translated to "near kidneys" (ad - near; renes: kidneys). The glands are part of the wider endocrine system which ensures that the release of hormones within the body is organized correctly and works as efficiently as it can. As small as these glands are, they are two of the most important organs your body has in its arsenal of defenses against the stresses of life.

The outer part of the gland is responsible for producing hormones which your body cannot do without – these include cortisol, which is important in regulating the metabolism of your body as well as helping with responses to stress, and aldosterone which plays an important role in the regulation of blood pressure in your system. Furthermore, the inner part of the gland produces hormones which are important, but without which the body may still be able to function – these include adrenaline which helps you to react to stress, and is an integral part of the "fight or flight" response a person has when stressed – and so of course the importance of these should not be understated. We will discuss these hormones in a little more detail below, however the important thing to remember is that these glands produce hormones which are important to your functions, even when you are not under a period of stress.

Why are they adrenal glands important?

One of the primary functions of the adrenal glands is in helping our bodies to cope with stress, no matter where it comes from; such sources could include illness, injury, relationships, employment or professional life and more. By determining how strongly we react to stress that is brought about by alterations in the body or in the environment that we live in, the hormones secreted by the adrenal glands can help determine whether the reaction is "fight or flight," meaning that they might cause the body and/or mind to either deal with the source of the stress head on, or retreat from it. How we react to that stress is largely a function of these hormones, and if they're not working properly, then neither will our reactions be proper. In order to properly respond to the stresses of our daily lives, it is necessary, even critical, that our adrenal health, that is the health of our adrenal glands, be maintained as well as is possible.

In this example, whether fight or flight is the reaction can determine how we feel in a certain situation, physically and mentally. For example if flight is the response, that could lead to other feelings related to tiredness or mood change, whilst the fight feeling could mean finding oneself in a feeling of heightened energy and strengthened (and potentially with heightened senses in relation to what is going on around us).

Either way, these hormones are critical in regulating how we react to certain situations, and what the outcomes from particular scenarios are likely to be.

These instincts are the evolutionary result of primitive man's natural need to recognize danger and decide quickly how to respond to it, as well as to survive times when nature or circumstances caused difficulties such as hunger, weather extremes and other challenges to survival. In other words, they came from our distant ancestors, who might have to make a sudden decision on whether to flee a wild animal or stand and fight it.

Today, however, we find the same kinds of reactions that our ancestors employed to escape the attack of a dangerous beast or situation being activated by the some of the stressors of our modern lives. A difficult relationship issue (whether it be at work or at home with the family), financial difficulties, lack of sleep, poor air quality, reactions to allergens or irritants, the results of drug or alcohol abuse— any of these might cause one of the hormonal events we have been discussing. Whilst it is impossible to eliminate all forms of stress from our lives, so the systems that help us to survive them are still as necessary as they were for our early ancestors – however we can try and add some regulation to our lives to ensure we are in a stressed state for as little a time as possible in any normal day or week. .

If adrenal function is not within normal parameters, as is considered in the case of adrenal fatigue, then you will find that your body will not respond properly, and will not adapt itself to the effects of the stress you encounter. It is considered that such a scenario can result in certain physical and psychological problems, and these, in their turn, can become additional sources of stress.

Normal adrenal function is therefore incredibly important to keeping the body's responses to stress in balance, and to ensure that those responses are beneficial, rather than detrimental to your health. Hormones secreted from the adrenal glands can also help to keep swelling and inflammation to a minimum when we are affected by physical triggers that may range from simple allergies to more serious conditions. This is because they regulate several different metabolic processes, including how we absorb and use carbohydrates and fats, how fats and proteins are converted into energy, how fat is distributed around your body (especially around the waist and sides of the face), normal cardiovascular functions and regulation of blood sugars and gastrointestinal functions.

We consider the key hormones emanating from the adrenal glands in a little more detail below, though even if you don't feel the need to get too technical, you will still hopefully find that the actions in later chapters are relevant to you.

So let's have a little bit of a closer look:

Cortisol

Cortisol is an adrenal hormone that is essential to your body's efforts to maintain life and health. Cortisol has three main functions – these are: aiding the regulation of blood sugar level; and aiding blood pressure and blood circulation; and helping enable the body to react to stress. For the reasons behind the latter of those factors, cortisol is sometimes described by some as "the stress hormone".

Cortisol therefore controls or regulates the sometimes beneficial, but sometimes detrimental, changes that take place when you are exposed to stress. Some of these changes include alterations in blood sugar levels, which in turn may cause spikes or reductions in your insulin levels; changes to your immune system's responses to infections; higher or lower blood pressure; and other alterations that can affect your health and vitality.

Cortisol levels are not static, but literally change from hour to hour. Each day, your body goes through a rhythm which sees your cortisol levels reach their lowest points in the early morning, when you are asleep, and reach their highest around eight o'clock in the morning. These natural changes are a part of the normal daily rhythm for an individual, and are extremely important. To some degree, these levels can be regulated though of course this would be the sort of issue for discussion with a doctor.

Cortisol has two primary things which it underpins. Firstly, it stimulates the breakdown of protein and fat to allow conversion to glucose in the liver, and it is fundamental in activating the anti-stress mechanisms we touched on earlier.

It is therefore necessary to your health for your adrenal glands to secrete greater amounts of cortisol when you are under stress, but it is equally important that your body's cortisol levels and other functions return to normal as soon as possible afterward – this is because higher than normal levels of cortisol in your system for an extended period of time would not be good for your system.

The sad truth, however, is that in most of western society, we can find ourselves falling under so many different forms of stress each day that our glandular responses are activated over and over throughout the day – at a frequency which would not necessarily have been the case when we had been exposed to less, or different, stresses and strains in times gone by

Living in such a higher octane environment can, then, result in higher levels of cortisol circulating in your system. The implications of higher levels of cortisol can include, over an extended period of time, weight gain and other health problems.

However, lowered levels of cortisol, where cortisol is not produced in sufficient quantities, which we are principally concerned with – this can also lead to particular issues, and it is these that are beginning to be described by some as adrenal fatigue – in this case, prolonged lowered levels of cortisol can lead to sever fatigue, exhaustion, depression, weight loss and loss of appetite. Note, however, that if you are suffering from such symptoms then a trip to the doctor is the best option – this book is designed as an introductory guide with some self help factors built in – if you are having progressive or frequent episodes of the type described above, then the actions described later should help, and build wider resilience, but these would not be something which would equate to getting a professional medical opinion. .

Aldosterone

Aldosterone is one of the hormones produced in the adrenal cortex, the outer section of the gland. This hormone is vital in regulating blood pressure, and it does this primarily through helping regulate how much salt and water is retained in the body. It also affects the metabolism of fats, carbohydrates and proteins. With such important functions it is crucial to the operation and balance of systems within your body.

Aldosterone is controlled in the body through the functions of a group of other hormones that work together. This group of hormones is activated when there is a decrease in the flow of blood to the kidneys, which may result from a loss of blood volume or pressure during bleeding, or a decrease in the amount of sodium present in your blood plasma. Whatever the root cause, this can be a serious condition, and these hormones are present in order to help you return to health as soon as possible. Of course such conditions could be extremely serious and if you are showing such symptoms then again you'd be best advised to seek medical attention as the best route.

Other hormones

Besides cortisol and aldosterone, the adrenal glands are also responsible for the production of estrogen and testosterone. Together, these hormones are all absolutely necessary for life and a well-functioning healthy body, by regulating bodily functions and doing this, in particular, when we are under stress. Related to this, they can affect our mental and emotional health, contributing to how we feel about everything around us, and how we think and perceive our environment. When we feel depressed or "down in the dumps," it can be the case that these hormones are out of balance - restoring that balance is a necessary part of any treatment regime – and this can involve aspects of self help around managing stress, and having an improved diet and exercise regime.

A wide range of effects, including physical, mental and emotional ones, come from these hormones, affecting everything from the level of your sexual desires to weight gain and loss of muscle mass. This is because adrenal hormones are derived from the steroid family – these are secreted by the adrenal glands, testes, and ovaries, with the hormones transported through the bloodstream to various organs where they regulate various vital physiological functions. Of course these are exceptionally cpmplex systems and you cannot be expected to understand each interaction – the point is that a healthier system can support all of these functions well.

Good quality of life is therefore dependent on the functions of your adrenal glands, and your quality of life is directly related to the level at which your adrenal glands are doing their job. Anything you can do to improve these mechanisms is worthy of encouragement.

CHAPTER 2: WHAT IS ADRENAL FATIGUE?

Adrenal fatigue is considered by proponents to be the result of a condition under which your adrenal glands are unable to properly function as your defense against stress - that is they do not produce the hormones we talked about earlier in the required amounts to regulate functions related to stress. The adrenal glands are the mechanism by which your body reacts to different kinds of stress, regardless of its source. As we have discussed, such sources may be emotional, mental or physical, but the underlying factor is that you need a well-functioning system to be able to adequately deal with such sensors.

The syndrome that is referred to as "adrenal fatigue" is actually a group of symptoms that are considered to be attributed to when your adrenal glands begin to function at less than their normal effective level. The condition is most commonly characterized by a sense of fatigue or tiredness that doesn't go away, no matter how much sleep or rest you manage to get. Whilst such symptoms can be caused by other factors, as regards adrenal fatigue these would most likely appear most frequently after a bout of prolonged, intense stress; chronic or acute infections; serious respiratory ailments such as pneumonia, influenza or even bronchitis. However, any kind of regular, chronic stress, whether related to work, money, relationships, or any of the physical types of stress we have touched on, can bring on the condition. Of course the control of stress is important for a variety of reasons, and it is important to try and keep it under control. The good thing is there are many types of actions which individuals can take to try and keep their levels of stress manageable.

People who are suffering from adrenal fatigue may look and appear completely normal, and may even seem to be the picture of perfect health. However, even though they often show no visible signs of illness, they may well be prone to complaining often of being tired, rundown or generally feeling unwell. In addition, they may depend on high levels of legal stimulants such as caffeine or energy drinks to motivate themselves in the morning, and in some cases even to stay alert throughout the day. Of course such symptoms are so common that the makers of coffee and other stimulant drinks have built a multi-billion dollar industry around it, and yes—they know exactly what they're doing. It is thought that many of these companies actually maintain careful records on studies about conditions such as adrenal fatigue and other conditions that drain us of energy, as the information can be used to make their marketing even more effective, often targeting specific areas or groups that seem to embody concentrations of such symptoms.

Effectively, the condition relates to a reduction in performance of the adrenal glands. If the requisite levels of appropriate hormones are not produced in the correct amounts then the desired response functions of the body will not take place.

The under functioning of the adrenal glands can be destructive to the lives of those who suffer from it, but there are actions which can be taken to improve the resilience of the wider systems, including the adrenal glands.

CHAPTER 3: CAUSES ADRENAL FATIGUE?

We have already introduced the concept that stress is the trigger for much of the work required to be carried out by the adrenal glands. We have explored too, the concept that increased frequency, levels or extent of stress can mean that hormone levels stay at levels, for a longer period of time, which might not be the case in someone who is under less stress. Such a scenario may have a retrograde effect on how efficient the adrenal glands are, and so affect the amounts of essential hormones which are able to be produced.

Stress can come from many different sources. It can be the result of physical or mental challenges, and could relate to work or home life. It can affect different people differently – and of course small elements of stress are actually required to prompt us to react one way or another, whether that is physiologically, or mentally. The issue is when stress levels are high over an extended period – this is something we are more used to talking about these days however, and further exploration of the issue is only to be encouraged. Regardless of the source of the stress, or whether it is a singular event or a repeated or chronic one, your adrenal hormones must respond properly in order to ensure you are able to react properly, and that you maintain proper health and wellbeing – that is that your mind and body are able to get back to a position of equilibrium quickly. If the response from the adrenal glands is not as robust as it should be, then you could be considered to be suffering from some level of what is known as adrenal fatigue.

In adrenal fatigue, it is considered that your adrenal glands still function; however, their responses are not adequate to maintain proper health because they are operating a lower level of efficiency in producing the hormones you need to regulate your body's reactions to the stress. This can be associated with a period of over-stimulation for the adrenal glands, which could be the result of a very serious stress event, or of a chronic stress that is so prevalent as to affect the adrenal glands' ability to function normally.

Who is susceptible to Adrenal Fatigue?

No matter who you are, you may find yourself experiencing adrenal fatigue at some time in your life. It affects men and women without regard to age, race or any other factor, and any form of stress, whether it be a serious illness or just an ongoing difficulty, can cause it no matter how healthy you are in other ways.

As with many other conditions however, there are things that can make it more likely to affect you. Some of these will likely be little surprise to you - and they include things like poor diet, heavy smoking, drug or alcohol abuse, lack of rest and lack of exercise. If you understand that these are key factors, then you are not going to be overly surprised by some of the suggestions later in this book as to what you can do to build the resilience of your system – however it is to be hoped that this book can act as a spur for you to take some concerted action in this regard. Please read on!

How common is Adrenal Fatigue?

Statistics on adrenal fatigue are not particularly easy to come by. This is perhaps no surprise as it is something which has been little understood to date – and some of the symptoms can be allied to other conditions. As we have explained, it is not something commonly referred to in medical books, and this makes it difficult to ascertain how common the condition is. However some reports from as far back as the late 1960s have suggested that up to 16% of the population could be considered to suffer from adrenal fatigue – or at least conditions associated with the adrenal glands not working to their full capability. This means that some take the view that when low cortisol levels, more generally are taken into account, then the percentages of those with adrenal gland related issues can be considered to be higher. It could, of course, be argued that the stresses and strains of modern life have increased by a fair degree since the 1960s – with the types of stresses now including more extreme events and threats from issues such as terrorism, economic problems and so on. In addition, the understanding of individuals about their own bodies has increased exponentially over that time too, and so people now understand much more about their own systems than they ever have in the past. They are also much better placed to understand how choices that they make themselves can have an impact on their health and wellbeing – and they are alos much better at being able to monitor that for themselves – consider the amount of table and phone apps, as well as wearable devices that are now available – all of these would have been unthinkable in decades gone by, but they al make for a more informed and understanding public when it comes to issues of health and wider wellbeing.

Are there health conditions related to Adrenal Fatigue?

As we have outlined, your adrenal glands are critical to the healthy functioning of your body – this means that they are required to ensure things remain in balance. The functions undertaken by the adrenal glands, as with other parts of the body, can come under more pressure in particular situations. These include increasing demands placed whenever an individual suffers from a minor or chronic illness or condition.

If you are dealing with such an illness, and you may often feel fatigued in the morning, It may be that you are also suffering from adrenal fatigue. Of course it is likely to be very difficult for you to make any sort of self-diagnosis. It is essential that if you feel you are having symptoms over an extended period of time, or witness particular changes in your own body, that you are checked out by a doctor – sooner rather than later if you have any concerns. The options suggested in this book are designed to improve the bedrock of your system by reducing stress, better eating and so on, but ultimately it can be for a doctor to decide whether your particular situation requires other changes, or medication.

How can I tell if I am suffering from Adrenal Fatigue?

The following list of questions have been put together to allow you to carry out a degree of self-assessment as to whether you may be suffering from adrenal fatigue. It may be that you can tick the box for some of these at various times, but we are really looking for a trend – can you say that some of these situations apply to you on a more regular or ongoing basis? If then you can answer "yes" to more than one of the following questions, and this is something which affects you regularly, then it may be that you are suffering from adrenal fatigue or wider issues relating to your balance and functioning of hormones – and going through the checklist is good for associated purposes – it might show up other factors which you can either explain to your doctor, or which you can use as a prompt to try and change those aspects of your lifestyle which can aid your health more generally. It might be worth asking yourself these questions a couple of times, maybe one day then another – as your mood might be different on different days for completely unrelated reasons (you got home from work late, the trash lorry woke you up, you were out later than normal).

So. having said all that, let's make a start:

Do you find yourself feeling tired at different times of the day?

Is it difficult for you to get out of bed in the morning, even though you went to bed at a reasonable time and got plenty of sleep?

Do you often feel overwhelmed?

Is it difficult for you to recover from an illness?

Do you often have a craving for salty or sugary items?

Do you feel that you are more awake or have more energy in the evening than you did all day?

If any of these things sound like what you're experiencing, then you may be experiencing a degree of adrenal fatigue, and you could consider implementing the suggestions in the next section of this book. If you are finding that you can tick a few of the boxes then you might also want to consider seeking some medical opinion as well as taking forward the suggestions in this book relating to diet, stress and exercise. The thing about an exercise like this is that even if you're comfortable with the answers you have given to the questions, then there is no harm in implementing the suggestions anyway, - for wider health and wellbeing reasons - so it is well worth reading on and seeing what you can set in train for yourself!

CHAPTER 4: UNDERLYING KEY FACTORS - DIET

Does the type of diet we are on affect adrenal fatigue? Absolutely; what we eat, when we eat and how we eat affects us greatly in many ways, including the amount of energy we have and our sleeping habits. So, let's take a look at some of the dietary approaches we can utilize to promote better sleep, increase our energy and support our adrenal glands. As with other lifestyle aspects, it is important to have a good understanding of what you already eat, and how it impacts on you. As a first port of call, think about checking out what mode of monitoring what you eat would suit you best – maybe noting on a physical calendar, using an app, or just plain old pen and paper – go with what works for you, but remember that in order to make changes you do need to have a good idea as to what your benchmark is – and you also need to be honest about this – don't "forget" to note down that doughnut or fizzy drink – in the end you are just kidding yourself (but of course you know that, enough of the nagging).

Remember that there are some foods that may help your adrenal gland health, and some that may undermine your system more generally, The former are not foods that are commonly found in American diets, but they are becoming popular enough in recent years to begin appearing in our grocery stores and restaurants

We have talked already about the importance of diet – it stands to reason that the way energy is taken into our body's systems is of critical importance. The nutrient and energy balance of the food and drink we take on board is fundamental to how well our mind and body can function –

but that does not mean that it is easy making the right decisions as to how to go about that.

Any healthy system needs a bedrock. The old adage of "you are what you eat" is true, and if you have a healthy diet then the chances of you remaining healthy more generally are also much higher.

A Basic Adrenal Fatigue Diet means an eating plan that is based on the common sense principles found throughout this book. Its purpose isn't to lose weight or reshape your body, but to help your body recover its health and return to normal functions. It's all about reducing stress, and ironically, this can't be "stressed" enough—in order to return to good adrenal health, you must reduce the stress that affects you, whether it be physical, emotional, mental or even dietary! A good, healthy diet will always help you move along that road to recovery.

Eating the right kinds of foods will give your body, and your adrenals, the necessary nutrition they need to let you function the way your body was designed to function. This means that you need to consume foods that offer genuine nutritional benefits, and this eliminates almost all processed foods immediately! Let's take a look at what nutrients you need, and then we'll examine the best way to put them into your diet.

Vitamin C is necessary for the proper production of the stress hormones, as are the B Vitamins, and particularly B5, also known as Pantothenic Acid, and B3, Niacin.

Also necessary is magnesium, which works like an enzyme that is necessary for the production of glucocorticoids. It also tends to calm the nervous system, and is useful in helping us manage and recover from stress. Stress can deplete your magnesium levels, too.

Zinc also works like an enzyme in the regular production of stress hormones, and also aids immune function. Any kind of stress can use up your zinc supply, but illnesses do so more rapidly than any other form.

People with poorly functioning adrenals often suffer from sodium deficiency, as well. This mineral is necessary to allow niacin to enter the cells, which is vital to our bodies' production of energy.

Tyrosine, an amino acid found in meats, fish, eggs, oats, beans, nuts, and wheat, is a component of the thyroid hormone thyroxin, necessary for proper thyroid function.

Consuming foods that are rich in these nutrients is important to anyone suffering from adrenal fatigue. Be careful about multi-vitamins that claim to provide them, though; many of these products don't actually have as much of them as they seem to claim, and it's far better to phase in a balanced diet, if possible.

Therefore, the first thing you must consider when you set out to deal with Adrenal Fatigue is your diet, because it is the single most important factor affecting your health. In addition, it is something that you can actively control. By consuming a diet that is designed to support adrenal health, you will be taking your first and most important step. In all probability, if you get it right it will likely cost you no more than your current diet (and often even less), and will bring with it a number of additional benefits, such as potential weight loss, a bolstered immune system and an increase in strength and energy levels. Associated with that you should find that your quality of sleep and cognitive capacity can improve if you have a healthier and more balanced diet.

When we avoid eating for lengthy periods, the adrenal glands have to work extra hard to produce additional cortisol and adrenaline in order to maintain normal functioning of the body. When our blood sugar levels drop for an extended period of time, it creates a stress reaction, thus setting the adrenal glands to work. Cortisol works to regulate blood sugar between meals and at night, while our bodies are at rest. Therefore, our bodies are in constant need of energy even when we are sleeping, and that's why it is important to eat in a timely fashion and to eat healthy meals and snacks on a daily basis. Of course the adrenal glands are on duty all the time – the issue we are considering is where the adrenal glands have to work at a higher capacity more often and for more prolonged periods.

However, it is important to establish the bedrock that we talked about previously – there is no point trying to make changes only to slip back into your old routine. That means that, in order to implement this new diet and take the first steps on your journey back to good health, it is important to consider a few key factors, and to lay down a few simple ground rules. These should help you keep to your plans.

As important as it is to eat the right kinds of foods, it can be every bit as critical to avoid eating some others. Let's take a look at some of them and see just why.

Fruits, including dried fruits and fruit juices, can increase blood sugar rapidly, so include them in a balanced way. Look for foods that are gentler on the blood sugar system, and eat these along with the fruits, to help keep it all in balance. Adding nuts, cheese or oats to a snack containing fruits can reduce the overall glycemic effect of the sugars in the fruit.

If you're eating as part of your adrenal fatigue recovery regimen, the how you eat and when you eat are equally as important as the things you eat. You should never wait too long between meals and snacks, to make sure that you keep your blood sugar out of the low range that causes problems and releases the stress hormones to try to bring it back where it belongs. This means that you don't skip breakfast, which really is the most important meal you eat each day. A healthy breakfast helps you to avoid blood sugar drops that can cause a release of stress hormones. If you don't want a big breakfast, a light snack is still better than eating nothing in the morning.

Then, eat several smaller meals or snacks each day, and set specific times for them, rather than eating the conventional three meal a day way that leaves you going hungry in between. That can cause the roller coaster ride for your blood sugar to go into high gear, and then you need the stress hormone to calm things down, and sooner or later your body begins to suffer more and more ill effects, until your systems actually begin to stop working. In general, you should never go more than a couple of hours without eating something that is nutritious and can help curb your hunger.

So, what kinds of food should you be eating? Apply some common sense, here, and it should be pretty easy to figure out.

We need to eliminate as many of the foods that cause stress as we can. Those include all processed carbs, like sugar and wheat products, all fast foods, all super sweets, like candy, cakes, cookies, doughnuts, etc. Get these out of your diet, and as hard as it may sound, keep them out! Indulging even once in a while will eventually lead to eating them regularly again, now matter how you tell yourself you'll only have one, at least for this week.

Now, we need to add in foods that are good for us. This would mean adding in things like lean meats, cheese, raw, unprocessed fruits and vegetables, good carbs that are gluten free, such as items from rice or spelt flour, shiritaki noodles, etc. Get the bad out, and the good in, and you're that much further along the way to a healthy adrenal system

So, what are the factors we need to consider, and rules we can usefully set?

Rule Number One: Avoid any kinds of food that will contribute to a worsening of your Adrenal Fatigue. This seems obvious, but in order to be able to make good choices around diet, then you must know what affects you in relation to the health and functioning of your adrenal glands – we will explore this in more depth later.

Rule Number Two: Consume foods that are known to aid in recovering from this condition – again, it is all too easy to say that an individual must strive to eat more healthily – but that means nothing if they are not able to understand what that actually means, and what foods can help your system be bolstered.

Rule Number Three: Develop a regular schedule for mealtimes – this is probably something which seems like common sense but often, with our busy lifestyles, mealtimes can be the first thing to go. Your body is flexible, but does need a degree of healthy rhythm to function at its most optimum. This probably isn't a massive surprise to you, but if, for example, you logged when you had your meals through a typical week, then you might find that it varied quite considerably day to day.

Well that all sounds simple, so far, right? It should, because it really is that simple; however, no matter how good the advice is that you find here, it will be useless to you unless you commit to following it! For this reason, we have chosen to add one more rule.

Rule Number Four: Accept the responsibility for your own health, and take this journey with a determination to achieve the health you know is yours by right! Again, this may seem flippant, but it is important to understand that you are in control when it comes to establishing the bedrock of a good diet for good adrenal gland function – and if you can manage this, then you will see the benefits throughout your system.

In relation to these rules then, it is important to try to identify any of the dietary factors that can contribute to bringing about adrenal fatigue. These can include underlying factors such as allergies, intolerances and sensitivities to certain foods, all of which can cause stress to your body – and so can make the establishment of that bedrock much harder. Such factors can act to interrupt the natural absorption and use of the nutrients our bodies require, and they can tend to cause inflammation and prevent proper rest.

Identifying and dealing with such underlying issues may sound complex, but actually it is relatively simple. Think about it this way - if you have a good idea which foods you're sensitive to, then obviously, you should be as careful as you can to avoid them completely – it may be that you have already made some steps in this direction. If you're not sure which foods you may be sensitive to, then you could begin by eliminating one of them for a few days and see if symptoms of sensitivity decrease. There are many aids available to help you do this – including online calendars and meal suggestions. Once you begin to really think about the foods you eat, you learn quickly what affects your body in a positive way, and you begin to notice changes in how you eat rather than what you eat. You may want to think about how you record these changes – a food diary, perhaps written online, could be a useful tool. When you have identified one problem food, then test another in the same way.

These problems can prevent our digestive system from doing its job, which is to make use of the nutrients we consume and then eliminate the wastes from our bodies. Because of this, some of the earliest signs of a food intolerance are diarrhea and constipation, and may include problems with eliminating waste from the colon. In addition, they can keep us from actively absorbing the nutrients in the foods we eat, which means that we will not be operating at our optimum energy levels, and can cause issues like inflammation of the stomach and intestines, which releases histamine. Histamine brings with it sneezing and coughing, adding further stresses to the body. Since they promote improper absorption of nutrients, our digestive systems can be subjected to the presence of detrimental bacteria, and this will cause a weakening of the immune system.

Eliminate processed foods, especially those containing added sugars like high fructose corn syrup. Many snack foods and sodas contain these sugars, and they are one of the most common contributors to Adrenal Fatigue and its resulting symptoms and conditions. Changing your diet must be a primary and critical part of your entire recovery program, and these simple suggestions will help you to achieve that goal.

whether they come from the fast food joint down the street or your grocer's deli section, rarely have any of the nutrients they started out with, and this is primarily due to the processes to which they are subjected. If it's precooked in any way, it's probably been through at least one chemical process or had something added to it that eliminates any benefit it may have had nutritionally. That means that when you eat it, your body has to expend an awful lot of energy just detoxifying the stuff, and that causes—you guessed it—stress!

In order to avoid this particular kind of stress, you should avoid refined carbohydrates. This includes any form of sugary beverage, such as soda, and anything made with white flour (in fact, most wheat products should be avoided), because they can cause severe blood sugar spikes. That can give you a burst of energy, but it will be followed shortly after by a crash, and your body's insulin begins to work. This is why many people turn to cakes, cookies and candy as snacks, to stimulate them with a blood sugar boost. The roller coaster ride of sugar spike, insulin spike, sugar spike and insulin spike means that the body starts producing cortisol at an amazing rate, just to try to cope with the stress that this practice puts on our bodies. Instead, we should concentrate on a diet of healthy carbs, proteins and fats that can be found in whole, natural foods.

Any kind of stimulants put a drain on the adrenals, and this includes caffeine from tea, coffee, chocolate and colas, as well as artificial stimulants like amphetamines. All of them will cause cortisol to be released, which then loads the blood with glucose. Suddenly, you're feeling a euphoric rush, but the down side is that your body immediately starts looking for the balance that it knows is normal. If it can't find it, then what happens is that your body begins to think the stimulant-laden blood is normal, and so the adrenals become less responsive to your need for cortisol. As a result, you'll find yourself needing more and more of your favorite stimulant in order to get the boost you want from it, and eventually it won't help at all. This is often why drug addicts find themselves needing more of their drug of choice; the body becomes used to it, and stops producing hormones that seem unnecessary while on the drug. Just like a drug addict, the best solution is to wean yourself from any stimulants.

One of the first tings you should do is concentrate on reducing the sugar in your diet. When you take in too much sugar for your energy needs, you are putting undue stress on your adrenal glands because cortisol is the hormone most involved with controlling your blood sugar levels. This leads to what we call "sugar crashes," which is the result of a spike in insulin, which then leads to craving more sugars and stimulants like caffeine to combat the resulting fatigue. It is a vicious cycle that will continue until you get a grip on your total sugar intake!

Also, don't think that just because you cut out the Frosted Flakes, you've solved your sugar problem! Snacks and junk foods are not the only sources of excessive sugars, but they are also found in things like fruit juices and other snacks and drinks that are promoted as being "healthy." The best sources of natural sugars are found in carbs like vegetables, beans, grains and whole fruits.

Consuming proper amounts of proteins are the best way to keep your energy levels where they should be, without resulting in blood sugar spikes or crashes. Beef, wild (not farm-raised) fish, free range chicken and eggs are wonderful sources. You should always try to purchase organic meats and produce, and you can sometimes save money by getting them at a farmers' market, rather than a health food store.

Fats are another necessary part of your diet, but be careful about how much fat you consume with meats. Instead, look into foods like nuts and seeds, avocado, butter, cheese and yogurt. It's important to get enough fat into your diet in order to keep your energy levels up and maintain your health, but you want to be sure that you get your fat needs from whole, natural foods.

There was a time when our ancestors ate every part of an animal that they could, back before you could go to the meat counter and get a slab of ribs. Our evolutionary grandparents consumed the meat, the fat and even the bone marrow, which is highly nutritious, and was even considered vital to recovery form an illness. In modern times, we've found evidence that bone marrow can reduce inflammation, boost levels of good cholesterol and even bolster and strengthen the immune system, so there is valid medical reasoning behind their primitive medical uses for bone marrow, and the most common and palatable way to get these nutrients into our bodies today is by making bone broth.

Bone broth is made by boiling bones (with or without meat on them) along with vegetables and herbs. While the flavor is excellent, giving this broth many uses in soups and stews, it is also an excellent source of minerals, and is proven to aid the immune system and improve digestion. Its high levels of magnesium, calcium and phosphorus make it ideal of supporting the health of bones and teeth, as well as your joints, hair, skin, and nails, because of its high collagen content.

Another food that you may not know much about is seaweed. These plants are known for high concentrations of minerals and nutrients that might not be found in your regular diet. They can be added to salads and other meals, giving any recipe a boost in flavor as well as nutrition. Many different kinds can now be found in many supermarkets.

When we have low blood sugar, it's natural to crave sweets. It's easy to reach for all the things that aren't really good for us, then, such as candy, cookies, doughnuts, soft drinks and coffee when we are fighting adrenal fatigue. Unfortunately, the energy that we derive from these types of foods is not the kind of energy we need, and doesn't last very long. Such a sudden spike in blood sugar, generating a similar spike in insulin levels, leaves the bloodstream so quickly that we can suddenly feel quite exhausted. This has become such a common problem that the process has become known as a sugar crash.

When combined with hunger, stress and exhaustion can impede our ability to make healthy choices. Most people just don't realize how serious the negative effects of excess caffeine and refined carbohydrates can be on our bodies. When we consume too much caffeine and/or refined carbs, it affects our hormonal balance, as well as severely interfering with our sleeping patterns. Many doctors recommend a gluten-free diet and a diet free of caffeine and processed sugars to those who are suffering from adrenal fatigue.

Not only are cortisol levels affected by adrenal fatigue, but our serotonin levels can suffer as well, bringing on tiredness. That doesn't always mean you need sleep; sometimes, taking a brisk walk outdoors or just engaging in some simple deep breathing exercises can boost serotonin levels back up to where they belong and eliminate the lack of energy.

In preparing your healthy, nutritious meals and snacks, use fresh, whole foods that are preferably locally grown or organic, and most foods that are seasonal are good for you, i.e., Watermelons, oranges, grapes, etc. Most fruits and vegetables are seasonal, although mass transportation has made them available year round to most of us. You should include in every meal and snack something that contains protein, as this will help curve your appetite and cravings for caffeine and refined sugars, and it will help to stabilize your blood sugar.

It's very important to avoid foods that contain preservatives and foods that have added hormones, dyes, chemicals and artificial colors. If you buy prepared food, it is always better if you can get it from a health food store or a grocery store that carries natural, whole foods, and for those times when a craving sneaks up on you, it is always a good idea to have extra snacks made up and on hand.

There are some beverages that can help support and restore adrenal health, while some others do not, but actually drain instead of restore. Those that restore and support adrenal health are beverages such as herbal teas, ginseng and vegetable juice (with salt), like V8. The beverages that do not help, but on the contrary do the opposite, are alcohol, energy drinks like Gatorade and drinks that contain caffeine.

"What about salt cravings?" you ask. Salt cravings and adrenal insufficiency actually go hand in hand, and they are both related to low levels of the steroid hormone aldosterone. Aldosterone helps your body to maintain salt and water, which helps to maintain blood pressure. When cortisol levels rise, aldosterone levels will decrease and aldosterone, like cortisol, is influenced by stress and changes depending on the time of day. If aldosterone levels are chronically low, this can have an impact on your electrolyte balance. One approach to correcting this imbalance would be the intake of sodium.

One sure sign of an adrenal insufficiency is experiencing symptoms of light-headedness after leaving a hot bath or shower, or when you get out of bed. If this is happening, you should consult your doctor about the possibility that you have low blood pressure. A good way to manage these symptoms would be to add a good quality salt such as Celtic sea salt to your diet.

When implementing necessary changes to our dietary habits, we may often feel or get stressed, which certainly does not relieve the patterns of stress that are already depleting our adrenal glands. Do not feel bad if you veer off course once in a while. Feelings of self-disappointment that are associated with self-preservation are normal, so don't give up; just have a little faith in yourself and your choices.

Directly related to rule number four above - one of the most important factors when trying to change your eating habits and your body is knowing how to structure your diet to achieve what you want. This means thinking about food differently – not just as a comfort or commodity, but as part of your wider lifestyle. This isn't as complicated as it might sound, and there is plenty of help out there. Fundamentally though this means establishing a meal plan , which is far easier to execute than trying to make decisions in the kitchen – when you are hungry you may not feel up to making something in keeping with your regime – but if you have planned and shopped ahead for it (or even made it ahead of time) then those choices are far easier. There are different ways to set up your individual meal plan, however it is important to benchmark your position before starting on your changes.

So, what does a healthy meal rhythm look like? By timing our meals, and eating healthy meals/snacks in the appropriate proportions, we can help our bodies to regulate cortisol and its natural cycle. You want to eat your larger meals early in the day, so that you have enough food store to be converted into energy and this helps in natural ways to maintain cortisol levels, while at the same time giving you more energy, so you aren't feeling so wiped out and drained throughout the day. You would eat smaller, lighter meals at the end of the day this will give your body the proper nutrients it needs for the time you are sleeping and it also helps to keep your body's natural hormonal balance in proper condition, where it belongs.

First, eat your meals at the appropriate times. Don't be like so many others, who ignore breakfast, grab a fast food value meal (or worse) at lunchtime and pig out like there's no tomorrow late at night! Try to establish proper eating habits, and they must include eating at the right times.

Breakfast, for anyone with adrenal fatigue, truly is the most important meal of the day. In most cases, when you sit down to eat breakfast, you've been fasting for about twelve hours (break + fast = breakfast!). Your body is in need of its primary fuel for the day ahead, and it needs a proper fuel that will carry it through the entire morning without cravings or hungers, so you need to eat a good source of quality protein, plus a small quantity of good carbs. You can opt for an omelet or a couple of poached or hard-boiled (not fried) eggs with some fruit on the side, or a nice smoothie made with milk, fruits and perhaps some protein powder supplements. Either way, you're getting the kinds of nutrients your body needs, and this is critical to starting your day off right! The thing you want to avoid is eating the kind of breakfast that most Americans think is normal: sugared cereals, pancakes with syrup, waffles and such are almost guaranteed to put stresses on your body that will cause even more problems.

Breakfast genuinely is the most important meal of the day. Even though we know it's important, it is really hard to eat when we don't feel hungry. However, eating a nutritious breakfast that includes protein will help balance your cortisol levels and metabolism throughout the day. It also helps us to feel less hungry at other meals, which keeps us from overeating just to make up for the lack we feel from skipping out of breakfast.

So, try to eat a good breakfast within an hour of getting up, as this will help restore blood sugar levels that were depleted while you were sleeping. Have a healthy snack around 9:00 am or so and try to eat lunch sometime between 11:00 am and noon; this will help prevent a large drop in your cortisol levels. Then, around 2:00 pm or 3:00 pm, eat a healthy snack, as this will help offset the natural cortisol drop that occurs around this time.

Around 5:00 pm or 6:00 pm, eat a light dinner. It may seem a little hard at first, trying to eat less in the evening time, but eventually your body will get used to it. Last, but not least, we can have a light nutritious snack about an hour before bed time, but be careful to stay away from and avoid refined sugars. Things like fresh fruit and cheese are really good choices, providing your body with the nutrition it needs to carry it through the fasting that naturally occurs when you sleep.

By carefully spacing out the meals and snacks we eat, we'll be able to avoid any extreme drops in blood sugar levels, and to maintain the natural functioning of our bodies. Our adrenals won't need to work quite so hard in order to produce cortisol, and can put their energies into performing some of the other important functions that we depend on them for. This will lead to having considerably more energy and personal happiness throughout the day!

Hydration

A further factor to bear in mind in this diet is hydration – proper levels of hydration are absolutely critical to all our bodily functions – not least cognitive ability and digestive function. Without proper hydration, the body loses energy very quickly and it's unlikely to survive more than three days without any water. Drinking enough water is vital to having a healthy body. Water makes up the largest percent of what our bodies are made of, so it makes sense that we should consume a good amount of it in order to stay healthy. If you are to be eating properly, then you must also be drinking properly. Directly related to this is what you may be drinking that is acting to dehydrate you – traditional tea, coffee and alcohol all acts to dehydrate – but there are so many alternatives on the market that you do not need to have to give up your routine of a hot drink at certain times of the day, and you can try to lessen your alcohol intake by replacing with soft drink options. Perhaps get yourself a soft drink cocktail book and see if you can make things a bit more interesting at home. Try also to have water with you when you leave the home – it is important to stay hydrated throughout the day and you may find it benefits you in relation to staying concentrated – often an issue even when in a sedentary occupation, where you may be looking at a computer screen or papers through the day.

Drinking coffee, tea and other caffeinated beverages can make you feel good for a little while, but they always compound the stresses you are putting on your adrenal glands. Caffeine causes adrenaline and cortisol to be produced in your body in precisely the same way they are produced when you suddenly find yourself in danger. The more often this happens, the more depleted your adrenal glands become, and so their responses to your stresses are not as robust as they should be. Additionally, it has been found that those who suffer from Adrenal Fatigue tend to feel that caffeine holds no benefit for them, and even coffee cannot help them get the morning energy they need. This is primarily because their adrenals are already so depleted that they cannot properly react to a stress threat.

Walking away from that morning cup of coffee, tea or soda may be frightening, but the damage they do to your system should scare you a lot worse! Eliminating caffeine from your diet may be one of the most important parts of your journey back to adrenal health. You may suffer some form of withdrawal symptoms for a time, but they almost always pass within a few days, perhaps a week, and once you have gotten caffeine out of your system, you will probably find that you feel even more energetic during your day; most who suffer from Adrenal Fatigue have indicated that they feel a balanced, even level of energy, and don't seem to have the crashes they experienced when using caffeine so heavily.

How hard is it to understand that you must keep yourself hydrated? It makes no difference who you might be, keeping yourself hydrated is absolutely necessary to good health, and it becomes doubly so when you are trying to recover from Adrenal Fatigue. It might even benefit you more to add a bit of sea salt or lemon to your water, since many who have Adrenal Fatigue syndrome also exhibit deficiencies in electrolytes and minerals that are necessary.

Adrenal fatigue syndrome, even though it has been recognized and treated for decades by doctors, is not recognised as a medical condition in medical books, so a lot of doctors don't recognize it today, even though it was recognized as much as a potential issue fifty years ago. Part of the problem is that there are conditions with similar symptoms, like hypoglycemia and depression, that can actually be caused or made worse by issues with the adrenals that sometimes fail to show up in the standard hormone tests. A lot of medical practitioners don't spot the adrenal connection, meaning that the patient won't get better, or his recovery may be slowed due to the fat that the adrenal problem is not dealt with as it should be.

Fortunately, lot of the most troublesome symptoms of adrenal fatigue can be made bearable by maintaining an adrenal fatigue diet, as well as making some very necessary lifestyle and attitude changes.

Understanding the physical effects of hormones will give you a grip on how any deficiency can leave you feeling drained, reduce your resistance to illness and food cravings, and show you clearly why following a valid adrenal fatigue diet can be critical to your health and recovery. As we've discussed previously, cortisol works with insulin to keep blood sugar levels where they should be, by helping the liver in converting glucagon, which is the fancy name for stored food energy, to glucose, the active form of sugar that we use to provide energy when we need it. Insulin, when it's working properly, causes glucose to enter our bodies' cells to provide that energy. If not enough cortisol is available, our cells can't get sufficient glucose, which means that your blood sugar drops to dangerously low levels that may even lead to hypoglycemia. That means not enough energy and a feeling of fatigue, and then we feel cravings for sweets or snacks that will bring blood sugar back up, and the cycle begins again. These swings in blood sugar levels can lead to more cravings, rapid weight gain, potential insulin resistance and, sooner or later, to Type II diabetes.

It's not a big surprise, then, that a proper adrenal fatigue diet might help to speed that recovery. In fact, when we take a good look at an adrenal fatigue diet, we see that preserving energy and controlling the stress response amounts to little more than sensible self-care. There is nothing to lose in starting and maintaining an adrenal fatigue diet and lifestyle, especially when you believe that your adrenal function may be suffering. When stresses pile up, the adrenals begin to be overworked, and that's when things can get hairy. That's when a good balanced diet becomes critical to ensure your adrenals get the nutrients they need to produce your stress hormones as you need them.

Besides the importance of getting a sufficient amount of the right nutrients, it's equally important to avoid the wrong foods. By developing a proper attitude towards stress and diet, you can limit the damage you suffer and put yourself on the road to full recovery from this condition.

CHAPTER 5: KEY UNDERLYING FACTORS - STRESS

Adrenal fatigue is thought to be directly linked to the levels of stress we have in our lives.

The good news is that adrenal fatigue is both treatable and curable. There are many things we can do to treat and cure adrenal fatigue for ourselves. The first thing is to decrease the level of stress in our lives. Granted, that's often easier said than done, you say, but the truth is that it isn't really all that hard. A lot of the time, we, ourselves, are the reason for the majority of stress we have in our lives. If we could simply adjust the way we respond emotionally to things that cause us stress, the resulting reductions of its effect on us would make all the difference in the world.

As we've mentioned previously, adrenal fatigue usually happens in response to something like extremely stressful circumstances or an extended period of even mild stresses, if they last long enough or happen over and over.

In such cases, the adrenals may have been working overtime for long periods, to help you handle the situations. When any major release of hormones is mixed with little or no time to recover, a poor diet, too many stimulants and little or no attempt at liver detoxification, the adrenal glands may not be able to produce enough stress hormones, even if they've been doing just fine for all these years.

What all this boils down to is that stress hormones are responsible for getting us up and going in the morning and helping us fight off the common cold or an injured limb, but they're also responsible for the ways we respond to other forms of stress, as well.

The reaction that we call the "fight or flight response" is the reaction we have to a perceived threat or danger, which tells us whether to put up a fight or run like mad. In our ancestors, it meant the difference between life and death when they faced a wild animal, an invading tribe, or a raging forest fire; to us, it means we treat everyday stresses like they are those exact dangers.

The sudden release of these hormones causes an increase in blood pressure, lung function, muscle function and our levels of blood sugar. At the same time, our blood vessels contract in different parts of our bodies, our immune response and digestive systems slow down, sexual interest fades and our bladders and sphincters become relaxed. All of this prepares us for the kind of vigorous physical activity that fighting or escaping in a hurry might require of us. The problem with us human types is that we can't always tell the difference between life threatening physical stresses and emotional or physical stresses, so that all of them can cause the same kind of response.

The important thing to understand is that when we mention stresses, we are talking about far more than just the physical kind. Mental and emotional stresses can cause stress hormones to be released, just the same as when physical stresses, like infection or injury, are present. When it comes time for the pounding heart produced by our catecholamines and glucocorticoids, our bodies can't really tell the difference between emotional and physical stresses. Being stressed out seems to be a normal part of modern life, with jobs, families, bills and so many other things that occupy our hours. We have to always make ourselves available to friends and employers cell phones, Facebook, email and so many other methods that it's almost more than we can hope to keep up with, and Heaven help us if we aren't right on top of whatever our families are up to all the time! Is it any wonder that a number of clinical studies show that we've experienced a drastic increase in anxiety and depression levels over the last twenty years or so?

Don't fail to understand the detrimental effect of all this seemingly endless stress on your body. Your adrenal glands are right out there in front, dealing with modern life in the this fast paced, technologically advanced century, and so a legitimate adrenal fatigue diet can aid your body in coping with all that you have to deal with on a daily basis.

Even though all of us have to deal with stress every day, including both the negative and positive types of stress, some of us are far better at handling these stressful situations than others, and at times, the only difference is in how we perceive the events that trigger the stress. One person might see a fairly common situation as being overwhelmingly negative, while someone else will see that same situation as a challenge that he finds exciting. All do us have been raised differently, and so we all develop different attitudes and skills in coping with different types of situations. In addition, each of us may find that we handle things differently because of genetics, or possibly because of our choices in lifestyle.

No matter what the reasons, even a lot of the folks who seem to be able to just handle anything that happens may be at risk of suffering from adrenal fatigue at some point in their lives, if they have enough stress, or have stresses long enough for it to affect them. Under certain combinations of stress, poor diet and over use of stimulants, adrenal fatigue, no matter how healthy you may think you are, will come to sit on your doorstep sooner or later, without a doubt. We all have a limit when it comes to coping with stress; it's simply that some people find theirs sooner than others.

How does "fight or flight" work?

First, within just a few seconds after we perceive danger, the adrenals secrete adrenaline and noradrenaline. These hormones can make you sweat, start to tremble and feel anxious. Your bladder and bowels may suddenly let go, and your appetite might vanish suddenly.

Next, the glucocorticoids kick in within minutes, and their effects can last for hours. These hormones suppress digestion and production of estrogen, progesterone, testosterone, human growth hormone and insulin. They immediately strengthen your muscles, including the heart, and raise your blood pressure to help you deal with whatever threat you may be facing at the time.

Naturally, because of the situation and the presence of these hormones, sexual interest pretty much disappears for the moment. Your blood sugar levels may experience a sudden surge, giving you a boost of energy to help you cope with whatever the crisis is, especially since insulin suddenly is reduced. The immediate effect of extra sugar suddenly flowing your blood stream can almost feel like a high, at least until things calm down and insulin starts to work again. It's absolutely necessary that you learn to live a life that reduces the amount of stress you experience, or else you must find a way to manage the stresses that you do face. You need to make sure that no kind of stress can make you lose your cool regularly, if you want to limit the damage that stress can do to your health.

That being said, if it's just not going to be possible for you to get out of your stressful job, or rectify a family situation, then you have to find a way to deal with it. You can accomplish this by altering how upsetting you allow these factors or people to be. In this way, you can make an incredible difference in the burden placed on your adrenal glands.

Again, all of this is about you taking control of what you can – it might be that you try yto explore methods which can help to keep you calm in those stressful situations in which you find yourself.

Cortisol is also helpful in maintaining blood pressure, but an excessive amount can lead to high blood pressure, while too little can cause the opposite, bringing on low blood pressure. This is one of the reasons that sufferers of adrenal fatigue syndrome are known to have low blood pressure and dizzy spells, especially when rising from a seated position, or getting out of, for example, a hot bath. Falls have happened that resulted in serious injuries, just because someone got dizzy getting out of the hot tub!

Cortisol helps to maintain proper heart functions, by regulating the balance of electrolytes and aiding muscle strength and endurance. If you're suffering from high levels of cortisol, you may feel heart palpitations, but if your levels are too low, your heart can literally stop. Fortunately, that is a very rare effect of adrenal fatigue that affects very few people.

All sources of stress cannot be eliminated, of course, but we can take steps to reduce our exposure to situations which cause it in our lives. Whilst we have touched on this a little earlier, this book is not primarily about stress reduction, and there are already many great books and online resources on the topic, however it is important to remain aware of the most important things we can do to reduce our stressors, and thereby seek to reduce the amount and effects of chronic inflammation.

A) **Psychological Stress**: The first step to reducing your psychological stress means reducing the things that cause it, plain and simple. There can be many such sources of stress – these may relate to your work (either paid or unpaid), relationship and family status, finances or health. If you find that your job is causing you stress (and whose doesn't?), then you have a variety of choices to improve the situation. You might want to think about whether you might be able to open up a line of conversation with your employer which allows them to understand just what it is about your job that causes you stress – it might be that there are some simple measures which can be taken to reduce job related impacts on you – and who knows, you might find that you agree there are better and more productive ways to go about things. After all, it is in the interests of your employer that you are as fit and healthy as you can be.

A more comprehensive option is to think about whether you could change jobs – this might seem like a drastic step to take, but who knows, it might be the very thing you have been needing to do for a variety of reasons. An alternative is to think about how you react to your job or learn to reduce stress through alternative means.

You might look to change your working practices – maybe you could work from home a day a week – cutting out a commute, or even giving you some peace to get key pieces of work done. If this is not an option, think about how you can build some exercise into your day, either by including walking as part of your commute, or something you do at break or lunch times – you might even be able to persuade colleagues to do similar, widening the benefits. Alternatively you could take up a hobby after work that will let you get your mind off of the job – maybe you could learn meditation or yoga and adapt the relaxation techniques that they bring to help you get rid of the stress of your job. For the most part, this advice relates primarily to paid roles. It might be that your principal role is that of a carer, for children, or for another relative or friend. In these situations, you cannot simply "change jobs" but there are likely to be conversations you can have with those closest to you to help reduce your stress levels in your day to day life. In some cases that might be the people you care for, but more likely it will be with others around you who may be able to take some of the load, or can help you devise easier ways of meeting your responsibilities – or they can just give you a break, plain and simple.

As well as the world of work, paid or unpaid, psychological stress can come from many other sources, such as family or other relationships, hobbies, and even a feeling of having unfulfilled dreams and ambitions and so on – whatever your position, you are able to regain a sense of control – but it might take a little time for you to feel that way. Whatever the underlying reason, in each case, once you have identified the source of the stress, you can find a way to cope with it that reduces its effects on your body. Whilst that sounds trite, the idea that we outlined earlier, relating to keeping a diary related to stress is often a good first step. Isolate the causes of stress for you and you can begin to take control and deal with them.

B) **Physical Stress**: This is a different type of stress, and for some it can be just as tricky to deal with – but again support is out there, though it may take a little courage to take control. Some of us may find ourselves dealing with physical stresses from accidents or injuries that are not going to go away. There may be measures you are able to take however – perhaps relating to picking up that physiotherapy regime you were once so good at when you had a medical professional pushing you. Alternatively, you may be able to talk to people in similar situations to see if you can pick up any helpful tips. Again, it is worthwhile noting down when the physical stress you may be experiencing is most prevalent – this makes it easier to devise mechanisms to deal with it. However, once again, it is strongly recommended that you try to learn techniques to help you relax and escape the stress itself. For example, meditation is shown to help with chronic pain, as is yoga, pilates and other forms of low-impact exercise. Explore, try and have conversations around the issue and see if you can find methods that work for you.

C) **Dietary Stress**: For many of us, this is the single most common form of stress that we have to deal with. This is primarily because the foods we eat most, and many of the drinks we consume, in this day and age are not the foods our bodies are best designed to deal with.. Of course the building blocks for most of the food and drink we consume remains the same, but today's foods, particularly processed meals are often filled with additives and sugar that are designed to make them last longer on the shelf, taste better and even become addictive so that we will spend more of our hard earned money to buy them. – We know that whilst those additives can cause stress to every cell and fiber of our bodies all day long (and at night too)! All of this means that the single, most beneficial thing you can do for your health is to change your diet so that you are no longer putting these stress inducing foods into your system – how to do that is the focus of the remainder of this book. Read on to learn more about how to change your lifestyle and dietary choices to make yourself healthier and happier!

Monitoring stress

Keep a Journal

We talked earlier about the need to try and set a benchmark to make sure you accurately understand what it is you eat at the moment – in order for you to make decisions which can improve your wider diet, and so improve the resilience of your mental and physiological systems.

By the same token, it might not be immediately apparent to you what the main stressors in your life actually are. It might be that you are able to carve out some quiet time in order to reflect on when you felt stressed – either through a day, or through a week – but you might not have that luxury. In the same way that there are many aids available to help someone keep a food diary, then so the same apply when it comes to noting down when you felt stressed – and what you did about it to improve things, if you have managed to implement a coping mechanism. Of course you could marry your diet and stress monitoring, and also ally it to noting down when you exercised – there are some electronic devices that can certainly help monitor your exercise, and they allow you to input information on what you are eating and drinking – the advantage of such an approach is that some of the work is done for you, and you are able to sit down at a computer to examine trends in your own life – it is not so easy to do this using traditional methods of pen and paper – but if that is all you have available, then make a start – and work out your own system

Whichever method you choose for stress (whether it encompasses diet and exercise or not), writing down your thoughts and feelings about the things that bother you is an excellent way to deal with stress! It gives you a sense of control over the events and situations that cause you stress, helps you to look at your problems from a different perspective and often leads to finding a solution you hadn't considered before.

Taking the time to look over past entries to your journal will help you to analyze the things that cause you to feel stressed, and this will allow you to decide what changes you need to make in your life to keep those things from affecting you so negatively in the future. Furthermore, if you feel you want to explore some of these issues with another individual – whether that be a trained professional, a friend or a family member – if you have dome reference material to be able to talk through, it makes things much easier, but critically it places you on the front foot – it puts you in a position of control.

Sleep It Off

A human being can expect to be asleep for twenty to thirty percent of their life. This means that the quality of that sleep is absolutely fundamental to everything they do. It not only affects their mood, energy and ability to make decisions, how tired a person is can have direct and indirect influences on those around them – friends, family, colleagues, co-workers – but also those they just come into contact with more generally, for example other road or pedestrian area users and so on.

As with many issues related to the human body, it is just as, if not more, important to understand how we function as individuals, than to be super-aware of the academic and scientific theories. If we are honest, how many of us really take the time to appraise ourselves in relation to our own mind and body? Probably not many, but if you can explore a few simple questions around your own sleep function, in particular, then you may be able to make progress in finding ways to have a more restful sleep.

How much sleep do you get a night?

Not enough is likely to be your answer. In the modern age, this is typical, but it is unlikely you will be able to give a particularly accurate answer just by yourself. We will explore tips and aids to understanding how much sleep you do get (and its quality) a little later, but given you are reading this book, you are likely to have a sense of this yourself anyway. Perhaps, every night, you say to yourself that you must try to get to bed earlier, as you are aware you are not getting enough sleep, or you know you are to be up early in the morning. Unless you are lucky to be very strong willed, you may find that the opportunity passes you by, and you head off to bed later than you anticipated. Of course you may go to bed and struggle to fall asleep, but if you are in that position then it stands to good reason that you won't be getting as much sleep as you would like.

Maybe one of the reasons you are stressed is that you are worried about your appearance. If this is the case, then getting enough sleep is already important to you, but as we've already discovered, it aids in dealing with stress and strengthens the adrenal glands so that they can do their jobs properly. Mixed in with better exercise and an improved diet, and it is to be hoped you will start to feel all you can be, and comfortable with how you look.

Make sure that you plan your days and nights so that you can get the sleep you need, and you'll not only look better, you'll soon find that you feel incredibly better, as well. This sounds harder than it might be – if you have chosen to invest in some electronic equipment which monitors your exercise, and allows you to input information on food you have eatn – then you might find it also has the capability to monitor your sleep. These are remarkable appliances – they can monitor how long it takes you to fall asleep, how you have slept through the night – were you woken up or merely restless – the quality and time of sleep you had over extended periods, when you start to wake up, and when you are fully awake. Not only that, this equipment is able to plot your sleep patterns over a week or a month or longer, and you can quickly start to see trends – maybe they relate to getting more or less sleep at the weekend, or that you tend to be more restless on certain nights of the week than on others. You might find that soon enough you are hooked, and trying to better yourself every day on sleep, exercise and diet – of course don't fall into the trap of over-analyzing yourself – these aids are designed to help, not make you feel more worried or neurotic!

Engage in Talk Therapy

Some people spend thousands of dollars per year on psychotherapy, going to counselors and psychiatrists in order to discuss their problems and learn to cope. In reality, the greatest benefit of this therapy for many people is nothing more than being able to talk to some about their problems.

If you can find a friend in whom you can calmly confide your problems and stresses, you will quickly begin to notice that they just don't seem as big and scary as they were before. This is because of the "shared burden" phenomenon; once another person knows about your troubles, part of their burden is shifted off of you and onto them. Since it isn't their problem, they are not affected the way you are, but the simple knowledge that you are not alone in understanding what the problem is will make it seem less daunting to you.

Meditation for Stress Relief

Meditation, which can be something complex that you must learn from an accomplished Master, or simply the practice of sitting yourself down in a quiet place to think calming thoughts, go over the events of the day and consider how you dealt with them, or even just letting your mind drift while you relax your body, has been shown to have enormous benefits on health. It can ease the feelings of stress, reduce your blood pressure, relieve pain and fight off depression.

Taking twenty or thirty minutes out of your busy day to just relax may seem like a waste of time, but the improvement in your state of mind and physical health will make you far more productive than you were before. Try it, and I am certain you'll find it as beneficial as the millions who practice it around the world today.

We've all heard the old saying that laughter is the best medicine, right? Well, it's true, especially when it comes to stress! Taking in a funny movie, hanging out with friends you can laugh with, even reading the jokes in a magazine can all help to reduce stress, and the more you laugh, the better you will begin to cope with the stresses in your life. Grab the family, ind the latest family-friendly comedy and go for it!

Laughter releases endorphins in the brain, which elevates your mood, and when you feel lighter, you deal with stress better. This means your adrenals don't have to work as hard, and don't get as run down, so laugh loud, laugh long and laugh often!

A Time to Worry

Similar to Meditation, taking out a time to do your worrying can be a way to deal with stress. Sounds counter-productive, right? How can worrying help reduce stress?

It's all in the when, where and how of your worrying! Choose a place and time where you will think seriously about your problems,, and then go there and sit as comfortably as possible. Begin to think about each problem separately, and let your mind consider various ways to handle them. Most people who do their worrying on a schedule report that they can find solutions to most problems in a single session. Give it a try! Of course a variation of this is to try and do some thinking when you are out and about. How many times have we heard of the author or scientist who is wrangling with a great problem, or who has come stuck in the development of a plot – they go outside to try and clear their heads, and hey presto, the idea comes to them, perhaps when they are thinking about something completely different. You have to choose the mechanism that works for you, but by the same token, it is important to try and get some time for yourself, when you are not caught up by the demands of what other people expect from you – you really do owe this to yourself.

Avoid Venting

Griping about your problems may seem like a way to "let it out," but studies have shown that when you vent in anger or frustration, you aren't really dealing with the problem at all. This will only increase the stress you feel, and cause greater strain on your already overworked adrenal glands!

Try the Talk Therapy mentioned above, instead, discussing your problems while calm and relaxed. You might also find that rather than venting, exercise, whether gentle or rigorous, can be a useful outlet for letting off steam. Don't injure anyone in the process of course, not least yourself – but you will likely know your own limits, and what exercises in particular you can use to calm yourself down.

Get a Regular Massage

If you can afford to go to a spa now and then for a massage, do so, and as regularly as possible! Getting a regular massage can have a tremendous positive impact on your hormone levels, particularly cortisol!

However, if a spa is out of your budget, find a massage buddy! Trade off with someone you trust, be it a spouse, a friend, whoever! Meet up once a week or so and flip a coin to see who gets the first massage, then take your turn when it comes! You'll be amazed at the difference!

And don't worry if you're not a trained masseuse; the idea is to learn that your buddy likes in a simple rubdown, and then tell him or her what you enjoy. The trade will be on that will greatly benefit both of you, and you'll feel amazing after each session!

Get a Hug!

A massage might sound like a bit of a bridge too far for you, but hopefully you might be better predisposed to our next suggestion. This is the most natural thing in the world, but there is not enough of it going on – not least because some of us feel a bit embarrassed at the prospect.

We've talked a lot about the hormones that are produced to deal with stress, but there's another one that can help lower your stress levels. Oxytocin, commonly called "the Cuddle Hormone," is produced in the hypothalamus when you are involved in any type of social bonding (like getting or giving a hug) and sent to the pituitary gland, from which it is released into your blood. It is useful in relieving the symptoms of stress and anxiety, and just darn well makes you feel good! Grab a hug whenever you get the chance, and don't be afraid to ask for one from those you love! It will do wonders for both of you!

CHAPTER 6: KEY UNDERLYING FACTORS - EXERCISE

Diet is important in healing your adrenal glands when they've been so badly depleted, but equally as important are the things you can do that will help you change the way stress affects you. One of the most critical ways to build resilience into your system is to take a good and appropriate amount of exercise. This is probably no surprise to you, but such advice is reiterated in all sorts of self-help books and articles for very good reason. If you can strengthen your systems, including your heart and lungs, then you will increase the amount of oxygen flowing through your system, and that will in turn improve the functioning at a micro cellular level in your body. In that case then, this chapter includes tips will show you some of the most simple ways to make those changes in your own life.

Now it may be that the idea of a weekly workout may be something that is not in your current routine. There is no need to think that the expectation on you is likely to be for you to leap straight into a daily hard pushing exercise regime – indeed, if you have not exercised for a while then this could be dangerous, and it is a good idea to visit a physician, health or exercise professional to ensure you do not overdo things early on. Having said that, it can be easy to make small changes to your regime – could you walk to the store down the block rather than jump in the car? Could you squeeze in walk around the block at lunchtime, or even a few lengths of a swimming pool? The chances are, once you build in exercise to your routine, you'll begin to want to protect that time – and will appreciate the many side benefits that regular exercise can bring. It might also be the case that you can persuade a friend or colleague to join in with this part of your new routine – perhaps you'll find hat friends or colleagues have been thinking of starting to do something regular too – ask around – you might be pleasantly surprised!

So, you can start simply - walking is a good choice of exercise to begin

Exercise can be both mental and physical of course, and both can be important in considering how well you sleep.

Mental exercise

We have also noted that stress and anxiety can be factors in relation to your adrenal glands and their health. We know that people who have had long days at work or at home can feel very tired – this can often be because thinking, concentrating and so on require energy in the same way that any other human function does – and this can lead to levels of stress which, as we have already talked about, relates directly to the functioning of the adrenal glands and requires them to work efficiently.. This means that it is worth thinking through your regime – at work, home or on the move - it is important to take stock of your personal situation and work to find a better balance through your day – but above all, try and make sure you get enough sleep to allow your body and your systems some adequate recovery time. What we are really talking about here relates to your mental health – and part of the package of managing stress levels relates to allowing yourself the space to think through what makes you feel good – so, if reading, doing puzzles or listening to the radio help stimulate you mentally or calm you down, then try and factor in some time through the day for these – anything which reduces stress levels is good when it relates to a well-functioning system – so don't forget the mental aspect of exercise and good health.

Physical exercise

It is generally considered that the quality of life an individual can expect can be improved if they get a certain amount of exercise during the day. Research has found that certain types of activity in particular – yoga, running, biking, golf, lifting weights and gardening are associated with better living and sleep habits. Other types of physical activity – for example housework or childcare – are more associated with poor habits as they do not have such cardio-vascular associations (though are certainly still hard work!). Whilst it has been known for some time that physical activity links positively to a healthy lifestyle, it is important for you to find an activity which suits you – and fits in with the other factors we have discussed elsewhere - don't let this put you off, as the overall benefits of exercise are high for so many other reasons. Explore what is right for you - and build this into your wider planning for a day or week. As with diet it is important that any changes you make to your exercise regime are sustainable. This means that if you can find an activity you enjoy, but which is still giving you the benefits of exercise, then you are onto a winner. Exercise is good for the body and mind – if you can find a team sport, at a level appropriate to you, then you may find that the team ethos is something else you find you can enjoy.

The other thing to bear in mind is how you track progress. It is unlikely you will be able to build such a routine straight into a normal functioning week for yourself, but if you can build in elements of it, more and more each week, then you will it easier to build your week around your exercise, rather than the other way around – as you get into your activity you are likely to want to do more and more of it anyway – exercise can be addictive like that! If you are able to keep a log of what you do, you can also look back to see what sense of achievement you can have related to what you have achieved. Recording your progress may seem embarrassing or discouraging at the beginning of your journey, but you will want those beginning weights, measurements, and pictures later to show yourself and others how far you have progressed. You might want to think about starting a blog either publicly or privately – this really can be a wonderful method to keeping track of your progress. Alternatively, you might want to keep a journal either on your computer or on paper as another great way to keep track. If you have a smartphone or tablet, you will find that there are any number of applications out there that can help you to keep track – some of them even calculate how far you have gone on exercise regimes and so on – use the technology! Once you begin to reach your goals and notice positive changes in your body, you are going to want to be able to compare your new self to your previous self. Always record your progress, no matter how small it may seem. This can help keep you on track to achieving your goals and help motivate you along the way.

Join a Yoga Class

Exercise plays an important role in your recovery, but for many of us, the thought of jogging, swimming, cycling or weight-lifting just isn't all that appealing, or we are not able to fit it into our daily or weekly routines for whatever reason. For those of you who feel that way, or have such constraints, I strongly recommend you consider enrolling in a yoga class.

Yoga is a very relaxing form of exercise, and while it can get you in shape and keep you there, its greatest benefit is in helping you to deal with the stresses in your life.

In addition, it has been shown to lower inflammation in the body, which further reduces the stresses you must cope with. Inflammation, which is actually an immune response which can aid in combating infection, has been linked to numerous health problems, including heart disease, depression and asthma.

Yoga is a hobby that helps lower stress levels and improve bodily processes simply by refocusing energy and distracting your mind from the various issues it goes over repeatedly on a daily basis.

One great way to work meditation and yoga into your daily life is to plan on a period of time where you can complete the following exercises and then segue right into your seated meditation session, thereby calming yourself and extending that period where you are focusing on physical sensations and being in the moment, rather than being lost in a mental list of stresses and worries. Again though, much better to introduce some of these elements to your everyday, and try to increase them as you go along rather than concede defeat as you don't have time to follow every aspect through. There are lots and lots of great resources available on yoga, both online and in books – have an explore at your local library or on yoga websites to see what might suit you and your circumstances.

For many people, yoga can become a way of life – something that transcends many other aspects of their lives – it can help them think more clearly, feel more supple, and help to strengthen their core areas – you might find you are hooked if you try it – that would be no bad thing .Bear in mind though, that you don't need to go to a formal class – you can try out many of the simpler moves in the confine of your own home.

Let's Go Walking

Exercise helps to relieve stress by reducing cortisol levels. Cortisol, as we've learned, is a hormone that is produced when we're under stress, like when you feel afraid or anxious or angry. High cortisol levels can cause inflammation and organ damage.

Exercise lowers cortisol levels, and this makes us feel better, leading to better health. A brisk walk can make a world of difference, and whilst it might seem simplistic, walking really is the easiest exercise available to most of us. It may be that you walk a decent amount already – if so, try to up the pace, or see if you can take a slightly longer route. If walking is not something you would normally schedule into a day, think about when you can escape your normal routine, even if only for a few minutes to get outside and go for a walk – all the better if you have some greenspace and fresh air to take in.

If you are someone who likes to go hiking, don't look longingly at your boots from time ti time – instead, be sure to schedule a nice long walk as often as possible, Whether it is a walk round the block, walking home rather than taking transportation, or a longer hike in the countryside, you'll be amazed at the effects walking will have on your body, and on your state of mind! All of this should combine to reduce your stress levels, and the pressure placed on your adrenal glands – all for the good.

CONCLUSION

So, there you have it. If you've read this book through completely, you now know what the condition referred to as adrenal fatigue is considered to be, its causes and effects, and how you can use diet and simple lifestyle changes such as diet, exercise and managing stress to start yourself on the road to recovery – and to improve your more general wellbeing – what's not to like about that? Of course for serious ailments, or issues which have been niggling you for a while, a trip to the doctor is recommended. Whilst the condition is not one that has been recognised in medical books and journals, it is something that is beginning to receive more attention, and there is no doubting the more general consensus that healthy and well functioning adrenal glands are absolutely critical to wellbeing and health. In these pages, we have considered some of the underlying issues relating to underperforming adrenal glands, and the types of things you can do – reducing stress, eating well and taking exercise – to try and give your system a solid bedrock on which all your bodily functions can rely. If you take some of the actions in this book, it is to be hoped that the benefits you accrue will go beyond the functions of your adrenal glands, and will leave you feeling more energized, better rested, and ready to face the challenges of life – both those you can control, and those that you cannot. Once you are able to take control of the underlying factors, you can begin to experience a better state of mind, and hopefully physical wellbeing. Good luck taking action, and here's to well-functioning adrenal glands!

Made in the USA
Lexington, KY
18 November 2017